# CANCER WINNER

A Brave Odyssey of Overcoming Cancer's Challenges and Emerging Victorious on the Other Side of Struggle.

Copyright © 2025

# Cancer Winner

All rights reserved.
No part of this book may be reproduced, stored, or transmitted by any means—whether auditory, graphic, mechanical, or electronic—without written permission of both publisher and autho except in the case of brief excerpts used in critical articles and reviews. Unauthorized reproduction of any part of this work is illegal and is punishable by law.

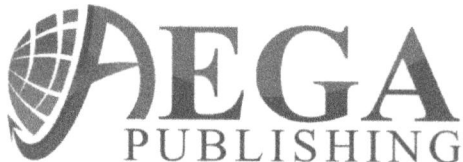

AEGA Design Publishing Ltd. United Kingdom
info@aegadesign.co.uk
www.aegadesignco.uk

ISBN 978-1-0685398-7-9 (Paperback)
ISBN 978-1-0685398-8-6(Ebook)

First Paperback Edition 2025

Printed in USA
**Norman Ceasar**

## Dedication
# My Uncle Wilbert Edwards

## Author's note
## Cancer Winner

Writing this book has been a labor of love. It has reinforced in me the importance of my health, to not take life for granted, but to continue to take care of me. My hope is that other men will read my story, see the importance and benefits of getting yearly check-ups. Taking control of your health it could save your life. I did and it saved mine! Just do it!!

# Contents

Introduction: .................................................................. 10
Mr. Johnson's identity: .................................................... 10
First Clinic Experience: ................................................... 11
Dreaded prostate exam: ................................................... 11
Urinary problems: ........................................................... 12
Urologist Dr. Baptiste: .................................................... 12
Why for me Dr. Franklin is concerned! .............................. 13
Urologist Dr. White: ....................................................... 14
Interview with Dr. Walsh's: .............................................. 14
Interview with Robotic Surgent Dr. Kim: .......................... 15
Interview with Dr. Walsh: ................................................ 15
Interview with Dr. Knee: .................................................. 16
Thoughts on Acupuncture: ............................................... 16
Decision to perform open surgery: .................................... 17
Why Dr. Walsh was happy? .............................................. 18
Good points for me were: ................................................ 18
I had the worst feeling! .................................................... 18

My happiest moment: ................................................................ 19
Things I was worried about: .................................................... 20
Why Kegel Exercises Are So Important? ............................ 20
I was patient throughout the journey: ................................. 21
Why am I interested in running? ......................................... 22
Cancer doesn't mean death is the only option: ................... 22
Advice to you: ........................................................................ 23
Final Thoughts ...................................................................... 27
Acknowledgments ................................................................. 27
Types of treatments .............................................................. 28
Surgery ................................................................................... 28
Radiation Therapy ................................................................ 28
Hormone Therapy ................................................................. 29
Chemotherapy ....................................................................... 29
Therapy .................................................................................. 29
Immunotherapy ..................................................................... 29
Laser treatment ..................................................................... 30
Laser Ablation ....................................................................... 30
Photodynamic Therapy (PDT) ............................................. 30
Rates of anxiety .................................................................... 31
Disease Stage ......................................................................... 31

**Treatment Options** ......................................................... 32

**Individual Characteristics** ............................................ 32

**Fear of recurrence and progression** ........................... 33

**Psychological Distress** .................................................. 33

**Impact on Quality of Life** ............................................. 33

**Addressing Anxiety** ....................................................... 34

**Routine screening** ......................................................... 34

**Psychoeducation** ........................................................... 35

**Psychosocial Support** .................................................... 35

**Cognitive-behavioral Therapy (CBT)** ....................... 36

**Mindfulness-based interventions** ............................... 36

**Genetic Susceptibility** ................................................... 37

**Variants in the BRCA Gene** ........................................ 37

**Implications for Targeted Prevention** ...................... 37

**Implications of Targeted Screening** .......................... 37

**Prospects for Precision Medicine** ............................... 38

**Genetic Counseling and Testing** ................................. 38

**Research and Future Directions** ................................ 38

**Higher Incidence and Mortality Rates:** .................... 41

**Younger Age of Onset:** .................................................. 41

**Aggressive Tumor Types:** ............................................ 41

**Access to Healthcare:** .................................................. 41

**Genetic Factors:** ........................................................... 41

**Socioeconomic Factors:** ............................................... 42

**Biological Factors:** ....................................................... 42

**Awareness and Screening Practices:** ........................... 42

**Prostate cancer and massage** ....................................... 43

**therapy:** ......................................................................... 43

**Relieving Urinary Symptoms:** ..................................... 43

**Enhanced Sexual Function:** ......................................... 43

**Prostate Health:** ........................................................... 43

**Stress Reduction:** ......................................................... 43

**Safety and Requirements:** ............................................ 44

**Professional Advice** ..................................................... 44

**Medical History:** .......................................................... 44

**Informed Consent:** ....................................................... 44

**Comfort and Privacy:** .................................................. 44

**Frequent Monitoring:** .................................................. 45

CANCER WINNER
# I Had Prostate Cancer. What About My Manhood?

A Must Read for Every Man In America. and The Women Who Care for Them!

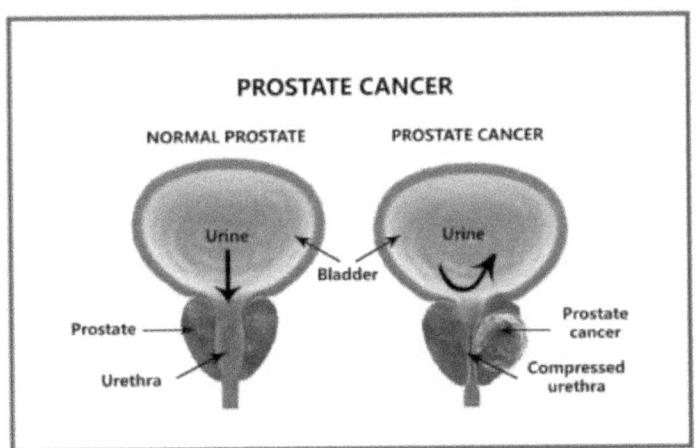

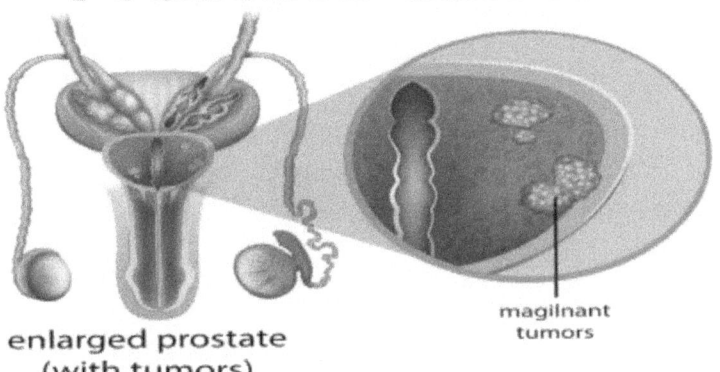

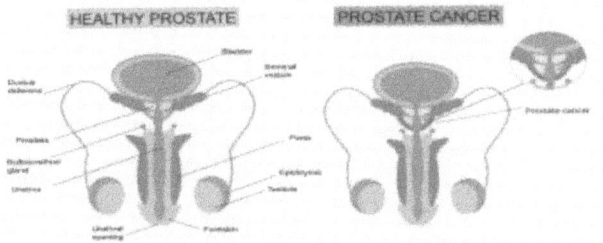

# Introduction:

The purpose of my writing this book is to educate men on how to beat prostate cancer, survive, and live a good long life. Consistent checkups and early detection are key. I dedicate this book to my uncle on my wife's side, whose cancer spread outside of his prostate gland. Unfortunately, he lost his battle with cancer due to late detection. This book has taken ten years to write and in those ten years I did something that you can too; I BEAT CANCER! I pondered on whether or not I should have the surgery, but after careful consideration I decided surgery was the best decision. So, at the young age of fifty-two, I went under the knife to have my prostate removed.

# Mr. Johnson's identity:

Mr. Johnson is the reason I got my prostate exam every year starting at age thirty-five. I was a Letter Carrier for the US Postal Service and Mr. Johnson lived on my route. Just about every day when I delivered his mail, I would see him working in the yard.

Most of the time he would be cleaning his paint brushes. He was an older man in his sixties, but he was still a professional painter. Still able to paint the exterior and interior of his client's homes. I found him to be a wise and practical man, who enjoyed sharing his wisdom with anyone who would listen.

One day while I was delivering mail to his house, we began to talk, like we did most days. Mr. Johnson knew I only had a few minutes to spare because I had a very long route, but this day I could tell he had something very important to tell me. I thought I had miss-delivered a letter by mistake. This sometimes happens, even if you are a seasoned Letter Carrier like myself. He asked me "Do you get a physical every year?". I said, "No I do not". "Why not?" he asked. I told him I didn't know, and never thought much about it. He said, " I bet your wife goes to the doctor". I told him "Yes, she goes all the time". "And your children" he asked. Yes," I replied again, "especially when they are sick". He looked at me with pain in his eyes and said "You should go to see a doctor every year to get yourself checked out you're paying health insurance, aren't you?". "Yes, it comes out of my paycheck once a month". He gave me his doctor's business card and told me to call him, make an appointment, and tell him that Mr. Johnson had sent me. The next day, I made the appointment.

# First Clinic Experience:

The doctor's office was at the Yeager Clinic in downtown DC. I arrived at my appointment thirty minutes early to avoid traffic, and good thing I did because there was a lot of paperwork to fill out. Once the paperwork was filled out, I was taken to see Dr. Miles. I told him I was referred to him by a current patient of his Mr. Johnson and I had come for a physical. Dr. Miles checked everything, and at the end of the physical he asked me if I wanted him to check my prostate. He said you do not have to have it now since you are only thirty-five, and it is recommended for men forty and older; but since I was already there, he gave me the option. I thought about it for a moment, "why not? Let's do it?" So, he put on a rubber glove and some ointment and felt my prostate. It only took a few seconds, then it was over. Little did I know, how true that statement would be? Every year thereafter, I had it checked.

# Dreaded prostate exam:

I know what it's like to feel anxious, nervous, and self-conscious about getting a prostate exam. Even though I committed me to taking the exam annually, I still had some of those negative feelings. To me, it was still "the dreaded prostate exam". The doctor would put on those rubber gloves and go through my rectum to feel the size and shape of my prostate. Man, it was the worst feeling. After all these years, I hated it still, but it had to be done. So, every year like clockwork I got my prostate examined on my birthday; but this particular the visit was a little different. I chose to have my exam at the Providence Hospital Wellness Center in my neighborhood. The day of my exam, I was nervous as always. I sat in the office, shifting from side to side, waiting for my name to be called. Finally, I heard the nurse call my name "Mr. Caesar".

I followed the nurse through the doors down a narrow hallway. We walked a little and then the nurse stopped, smiled, and directed me into an exam room. After the nurse took my weight and blood pressure, Dr. Jay walked in. To my pleasant surprise, Dr. Jay was a woman. I was relieved, to say the least. She made me feel at ease while she checked every part of my body, including my prostate with the well-known reliable "glove". I continued to see Dr. Jay for the next few years. I no longer felt the dread of having the exam and preferred Dr. Jay over my male doctors. My advice to every man dreading the gloved finger, find a female doctor to conduct your physical. It surely put me at ease and it might make your whole experience more comfortable.

## Urinary problems:

I remember what my body was going through before an exam that led up to my prostate cancer detection. I was having these terrible symptoms, and at the time, I didn't know what they meant. I recall having my sleep interrupted two or three times a night with the urgency to urinate.

As soon as I was comfortable in bed and sleeping well, I would wake up and go to the bathroom to urinate. I would disturb my sleeping wife who already had her issues with sleep and dashed to relieve myself. I tried everything, not drinking late, emptying my bladder before going to bed, but nothing seemed to make a difference. Then it began to get worse, not only was I having to repeatedly dash to the bathroom in the middle of the night, I began having problems with actually urinating. I was blown away. I could not understand how it was that I was losing sleep because I had to urinate, and then when I tried to urinate I couldn't. I could only produce small drops, and then to make it even more unbearable, I began experiencing pain. I would later learn that as the prostate enlarged, it would put pressure on the urethra vessel which carries urine from the bladder through the prostate gland.

## Urologist Dr. Baptiste:

Every year after my physical which included blood work at Providence Hospital's Wellness Center I would take the results to my primary doctor, Dr. Franklin, whom I had been seeing for many years, for his review, consultation, and prescriptions for my high blood pressure medicine. This time when he looked at my PSA numbers, from the blood work, he said to me, your numbers have gone up compared to the last few years. At that point, I was age fifty-one and my PSA was 3.0. He compared it to the previous years, and it showed my PSA numbers had gradually gone up. He said I think it's time for you to see a specialist or Urologist to make sure everything is okay. I said

OKAY fine. I have a friend, named Alan, who I have known for a long time who was being treated for prostate cancer with hormone treatments. He told me his doctor was very good, so I will get the doctor's number and call for an appointment.

I made a morning appointment to see Dr. Baptiste when I called him. His office was close to where I worked, therefore, I did not have to take a whole day off from work. I went to see him a week later. I took my medical records so he could see the progression of my PSA numbers. The first thing he wanted to do was to check my prostate. I thought to myself, here we go again with "the glove". Then I thought again, this is the way it has to be, if I want to live, I have to let professionals do what he is trained to do. When he checked my prostate, it was enlarged, which was not unusual for my age. The progression of my PSA numbers did not bother him at the time. He would be more concerned if they are 4.0 or higher. He said listen, let's take a look at your PSA numbers next year. Make sure they send your blood work directly to me so I can see them, then you can come back, and we can talk about it.

# Why for me Dr. Franklin is concerned!

The next year as always, I had my physical and PSA blood work done at the Providence Hospital Wellness Center. I took my blood work and PSA numbers to Dr. Franklin, my primary doctor, for review and consultation. My PSA numbers went up from the last year from 3.2 to 3.4. This concerns him because of how fast it was going up. He told me he wanted me to go see his doctor. He gave me a referral to see Dr. White his Urologist. He told me he call to let him know that I would be making an appointment to see him. I did not know what to expect after my talk with Dr. Franklin, but I knew I had to follow through on my prostate and PSA situation. It was my responsibility to stay on top of it, and get to the bottom of the problems that I was having. I could not put it off hoping it would go away or thinking I was too busy to deal with it right now. I made my mind up to stay on top of my health and make it a priority. If I did not, no one else would. I realized I must take the time to take care of my Temple, my body is my responsibility.

# CANCER WINNER
# Urologist Dr. White:

I made an appointment to see Dr. White in two weeks later. It was the earliest appointment I could get. The day of my appointment I was nervous. During my exam, Dr. White also found my prostate to be enlarged. He said that it wasn't unusual for it to be largely based on your age, but not on the size that mine had grown. Also, my PSA numbers were rising which was another problem. Based on his findings, he recommended that I get a Biopsy. He said although Biopsies are not normally performed on men of my age, it was necessary for this instance. He scheduled me for a Biopsy for the following week. He took twelve samples of my prostate during the Biopsy. When he called me at work the following week, he told me that a small amount of cancer had been found in one of the samples. He said "Don't worry, we found it early, you should be able to live into your seventies." I said to him "Dr. that won't work for me, I promised myself I'd play golf into my eighties!" Dr. White expressed his understanding and scheduled me to come in the next week to discuss my options. I was fifty-two when I received the prostate cancer diagnosis. The big "C" is not a word anyone wants to hear. The next week when I sat down with Dr. White to discuss my options, the first thing he said was "You should thank the Lord that your prostate was enlarged, prompting me to do the biopsy". He offered me a few treatment options such as radiation, implants, hormones, or surgical removal of the prostate that held the tumor. Removing the prostate was fine because I had no intention of having more children; being already the father of a boy and a girl.

# Interview with Dr. Walsh's:

On the following Sunday, after church service, I told my Pastor Robert G. Childs about the Prostate diagnosis and asked him for prayer. He not only prayed with me and told me this diagnosis was not unto death, he referred me to his surgeon at Johns Hopkins Hospital in Baltimore, Dr. Walsh. He said that Dr. Walsh was the best doctor in the field of Prostate Cancer, that was all I needed to hear! I got a recommendation and a chance for a second opinion. I contacted Dr. Walsh's office and made an appointment. By the time I met with him, he had reviewed my case and sent it to him by Dr. White, who did my Biopsy. During our meeting, he explained to me that based on his experience, I did not need to do the surgery right away. But he suggested that I not wait too long. He told me with African American men, the cancer can become a lot more aggressive. If cancer moves outside of the prostate gland, you could be in big trouble. If it gets outside, it could affect other organs within the body. He said, "Go home and think about it. Give me a call when I make up my mind to have the surgery". After talking with Dr. Walsh, I was torn between the need to have the surgery done and the thoughts that I was having – I do not have time for this - I have a busy life - why me and why now? After a day or so, I calmed down and decided I had to deal with the hand dealt to me. I felt it was important that I get this taken care of, but I did not feel comfortable with making a decision right away. I needed more information. I needed to do more research.

# Interview with Robotic Surgent Dr. Kim:

While reading and researching over the next week or so, I learned about Robotic Surgery and how it was less invasive with a shorter recovery time. I called Dr. Walsh's office, spoke with his receptionist and explained to her that I needed to talk to Dr. Walsh about something very important that had come up and would he give me a call? I left my phone number. I think it was the next day he called me back. He said, "This is Dr. Walsh, how are you"? I said, "I'm doing fine, but I wanted to ask you a question. He told me at that that he did not do the Robotic Surgery. He referred me to a young doctor, at Johns Hopkins, who did Robotic Surgery. So, I called the doctor, his name was Dr. Kim, and made an appointment to speak with him.

## Interview with Dr. Walsh:

This would now be the third opinion on my condition. You may notice that I didn't like using the "C" word when speaking about my condition. Did not want to claim it, but doing everything I could to deal with it. I met with Dr. Kim and he told me yes, he does Robotic Surgery and I would be a good candidate for it. But he felt that Dr. Walsh would be my best bet, especially since my chances of not being impotent and being incontinent were less likely. He further explained to me that Dr. Walsh was the best in the business. He trained him in Prostatectomy (Open Surgery), therefore he does both Robotic Surgery and Prostatectomy. In talking with Dr. Kim, I was even more confident that Dr. Walsh would be the best doctor to do my surgery.

# Interview with Dr. Knee:

I went back to Dr. Franklin, my primary for my scheduled follow-up. During my appointment, I shared my diagnosis and the opinions provided to me by the three doctors. He prayed with me, then told me about a friend of his who had breast cancer and how she opted to try acupuncture and she was cured. He said to me, why don't you try acupuncture?", 'give it a try, what do you have to lose, it couldn't hurt. I said OKAY because I didn't want to go through surgery anyway. I was willing to try anything. He gave me the name of the Doctor. Her name was Dr. Knee and her office was right in town. When I called and made an appointment, I explained to her receptionist that I had been diagnosed with Prostate Cancer and I was referred to her by Dr. Franklin. I was given an appointment for the following week. I didn't know what to expect. I never had acupuncture before. So, my wife went with me to my appointment. I was a bit nervous and did some deep breathing exercises to relax my nerves while I waited to be seen. In no time my name was called and I was taken back to a room. Shortly thereafter, Dr. Knee came in. I told her about my diagnosis. She said she thought acupuncture would heal my she stuck me with ten to twelve needles in my lower abdomen. The treatment took about twenty minutes and $200. She told me to wait about thirty days and go back to get my PSA done, and that I should be okay.

# Thoughts on Acupuncture:

I called Dr. Walsh and told him that I tried the acupuncture that was recommended by my primary doctor, Dr. Franklin. Also, I wanted to wait thirty days to give this a try to see if it would help me, because I was desperate. I wanted to try everything possible before I went under the knife, so I need the next thirty days to see if the acupuncture worked. He chuckled a while, and said okay, but I don't want you to wait too long. I am a very busy man. If I were to keep putting it off then he could not be my doctor. I said okay, I understand. I told him I also had another problem that I needed to take care of before having any treatment. I was in the middle of renovating a rental property and I would like to try to finish the renovation before scheduling surgery. I was a part-time real estate investor and had no one to work on this for me.

Dr. Walsh said he understood and that made sense.

# Decision to perform open surgery:

Well after waiting the suggested thirty days, I had my PSA done again and there was no change. I was still at 3.6. So, after all the doctor's opinions, my research, Acupuncture treatment and let's not leave out prayers, I chose the Prostatectomy (open surgery) to completely remove my prostate. I called Dr. Walsh and made an appointment to have my surgery done on November 16, 2006 at 8:00 am. The evening after surgery, around 5:00 pm, Dr. Walsh came into my room to check on me and to see how I was doing. I didn't expect to see him. I thought maybe he would send one of his assistants. To my surprise, he walked into my room and asked me how I was doing and feeling. I told him I was doing well. A little soreness, but other than that I'm doing well. I thanked him for taking good care of me. My wife was in the room with me when he came in. He told us when trying to remove my Prostate Gland almost broke his back because it was so large. He smiled, then said you are going to be okay. Everything went well. You did not lose any blood; therefore, we did not have to use the blood you gave a couple of days before the surgery. So, I told them to donate blood to someone else. Dr. Walsh told me I would be in the hospital recuperating for the next two days, after which I would be able to go home. He told my wife that he would call her as soon as he received the results from my Prostate lab work. I understand once they remove the prostate, they send it to the lab and put it under a microscope. For the next two days, I was treated well at the hospital by the staff. The nurses and the assistant doctors came by regularly to check on me. I even had a female nurse bathe me each day and she did a great job. I was treated like a king at Johns Hopkins and did not want to leave. Sure, enough on the third day, I was released from the hospital. As I prepared to leave, I said all my goodbyes to the staff and thanked them for a job well done. I felt like the happiest man in the world because now I was cancer-free. This was the level of my faith. There was no more cancer. I left the hospital with my wife. I had a catheter taped to my very uncomfortable leg but it was something I had to get used to it for the next ten days. It was part of the process to get me to complete healing.

# Why Dr. Walsh was happy?

On the way home I asked my wife to stop for something to eat. I do not eat red meat, so we looked out for a seafood restaurant. We found a nice little place to eat and had lunch. Afterward, my wife drove me straight home and helped me get into the house. All I wanted do was to lie down and get some rest. I had one prescription that needed to be lled, so she took it to the pharmacy. After she got home, she told me while she was out getting my prescription lled and shopping for groceries, Dr. Walsh had called her. The lab report was back and the cancer was contained in the Prostate Gland. My Gleason score was seven. That it was great news and what we were praying for was that once the prostate was removed, I would be cancer-free. Weeks later during a phone call appointment with Dr. Walsh told me he was very happy for me. The results from the operation worked out as we had hoped, by nding the cancer early. The cancer was inside the prostate and had not moved outside of it.

# Good points for me were:

I felt truly blessed that my cancer was found in its early stage, when it is most curable. My Gleason score was seven right in the middle, meaning moderately well dierentiated. It was not a low-grade cancer nor was it a high grade cancer. The Gleason score is a way to classify the severity of cancer based on the way, it looks under a microscope. Mine was right in the middle. This is why I stress the importance of having an annual physical and blood work with a PSA check. You do not want to fool around with this, because if there is cancer in your prostate you want to nd it as soon as possible. The sooner you know your PSA numbers and start tracking them the better.

# I had the worst feeling!

After surgery, I had a Catheter. The nurses showed me how to empty the bag attached to it and replace it. I stayed in the hospital for two days. I was sent home with the Catheter. I think this was the worst part of the surgery, having the bag attached to me at all times. Sometimes I would get muscle spasms because of the catheter. And it was very painful. However, it only lasted maybe thirty seconds or so, but I would have them a few times a day. I suppose the good news was I only had to use the medicine for my pain a couple of times. Thank God, I was never put on any other drugs. The catheter was only supposed to stay in for about ten days. However, ten days would have been up the day after thanks giving, but the o-ce was closed, so I had to wait until Monday. Therefore, the catheter was in three days longer than normal. My appointment was the following Monday and I got there early. One of Doctor Walsh's assistants snatched the catheter out, quickly before I knew it. What a relief that was.

Every day for thirteen days, everywhere I went the catheter was with me. I wore sweatpants to make sure I had enough room for the bag that was tapped to my leg. It was inconvenient especially when I went out for walks to get out of the house for a while or when I went out to check with my guys who were renovating a rental property that I started before my surgery. I had let him in the morning, go back home to rest, then go back in the evenings to check the progress of their work and lock up for the day. It was a pain, but thank God I got through it.

# My happiest moment:

Now fourteen years later, I am in the best health and shape of my life. I want to rst give thanks to Jesus Christ my Lord, for bringing me through this health crisis, and letting me know that it was not unto death. He orchestrated this whole experience of my life. He placed people in my life who encouraged me to get my prostate checked, and because I continued to get it checked every year, we were able to nd the cancer early. For many people, cancer is a death sentence, but I did not want to hear talk about death and dying. I wanted to be encouraged to live. When I found out about the diagnosis, I shared the information with my wife and my pastor only. I learned that my pastor had been diagnosed with prostate cancer the year before, and he shared his journey with me and which helped ease my uneasiness. He had said that Dr. Walsh was the best doctor in the eld of prostate cancer, that was all I needed to hear! I was excited to know that my "manhood" could be saved. I quickly contacted Dr. Walsh.

# Things I was worried about:

Dr. Walsh, who had vast knowledge and experience in treating Prostate Cancer, performed the surgery using the technique he developed called the Nerve-Sparing technique. This technique allowed him to remove the prostate gland without causing any damage to the nerve bundle that is responsible for erection and bladder control; and with that, Dr. Walsh performed my a very successful Prostatectomy. Though the surgery went well and he was able to remove the diseased Prostate Gland, Dr. Walsh warned that going forward, it wouldn't be all smooth sailing, but I would be alive, and likely cancer-free. It was 2:30 am when I awoke from surgery at John Hopkins Hospital in Baltimore, Maryland. I remember wondering what my life would be like now. How would the surgery affect me? physically? Would I be able to do and enjoy golf, tennis, and jogging? and have a fulfilling sex life? The surgery was done, the tumor removed, and I was finally cancer free. But now, I was faced with a new battle, a battle of mental proportions, a battle of self. As I look back on this, I realize, that because of Dr. Walsh's warnings, the process was tolerable. Smooth sailing it was not. It was months and months of incontinence, which meant I did not have full control of my bladder. However, as the months progressed, I gained better control of my bladder by doing Kegel exercises per the doctor's instruction. This exercise you can do before and after cancer treatment to help strengthen the pelvic floor muscle that controls your urine flow.

# Why Kegel Exercises Are So Important?

The Kegel exercise is one of the most effective ways to control incontinence without medicine or surgery. is the control over the starting and stopping of the urine flow? This is done from a standing position only. When you start to urinate stop the flow, hold it for maybe a count of ten, then release it and continue the flow. Repeat the process two to three times, as you feel the urge to urinate. Doing this exercise, daily throughout the day, helped me to control my bladder leaks. I was also warned by my doctor to be careful to limit my caffeine and alcohol intake as this worsens controlling the bladder. Therefore, even after fourteen years post-surgery, I continue my Kegel exercise and limit my caffeine and alcohol intake. Besides not having full control over my bladder, which the second most important thing that Dr. Walsh warned me about was that it would take some time to get your erections back. He told me not to worry, it would comeback. Just be patient. He had said from his experience if you had a good erection before surgery, then chances are you will have erections again.

# I was patient throughout the journey:

I was patient because I was confident that the decision to have the nerve-sparing technique, that he invented, better my chances of sparing the nerves that are responsible for the control of the erection and bladder. It required him to be very careful and delicately remove the prostate and not damage those nerves. Thankfully, a few months after surgery my erections got better and better. Not like pre- surgery, but I was back! It was a small price to pay to stay alive. So, you see guys, it wasn't so bad. I am enjoying retirement and my family living my best life! Some of my friends asked me if was I depressed while going through the diagnosis of Prostate Cancer and after surgery. One asked how did I not let it get into my head. They say they don't recall there being any outward sign that I was going through this challenge. I told them this may sound funny, but I did not have time to be depressed. I was determined not to let this inconvenience stop me from reaching my goal and enjoying my life. You see at the time I was planning to retire in three more years.

I was not depressed, because one day while my pastor and my church family prayed with me, I recall him saying this is "not unto death". I felt at peace because I was already speaking those same words over my life. Also hearing it from him, who had gone through the same surgery about eleven months before, gave me confirmation. It was my pastor who referred me to his doctor. Dr. Walsh at Johns Hopkins who also performed this same surgery on him. I was told he was the best and had already performed over 3000 of these surgeries. I knew with God on my side and with the best doctor in the business,in the middle of a house renovation.I knew I was getting better. Besides the doctor had told me he was going to take good care of me. I didn't have time to be depressed because I was in the middle of a house renovation. I was renovating one of my rentals properties and I had to stop working on it to have the surgery. It was imperative that I have the surgery and get healed sooner than later, so I could get back to working on thehouse. I needed to get it finished so I could get it rented. As a real estate investor, you cannot make money with a house is vacant. Renting houses is what I planned to use to supplement my retirement income so I can live the life I dreamt about. So, you see, there was no time to be depressed and feel sorry for myself. I just had to follow my doctor's instructions and keep it moving because I have a dream to fulfill. So, the first thing I did was set a goal. A simple, complex, achievable goal. Running was my life at that time and the thought.

## Why am I interested in running?

One day hitting the pavement again was exhilarating. I would run a 5k. If I could do that, I could do anything. The second thing I did was allow myself the time to heal properly. Physically over-extending myself would only forfeit my goal, and potentially interfere with my recovery process, and I wasn't willing to risk either. Once my body finally caught up to my mental readiness and I was completely healed, I began to train for my first 5k post-surgery. The training took my mind off of all I had endured in the recovery process and I was focused on one thing, running. A year later, I ran a 5k (3.2 miles) race in 40 minutes. It wasn't my best finishing time, but I did it. It was at that point; I got my life back. I would also like to contribute my physical and mental recovery to the dedication and the support of my wife of forty-four years, who helped nurse me back to health and went through this journey with me. None of this I could have done alone, I have had help, counsel and encouragement everywhere I turned and for that, I am truly blessed.

## Cancer doesn't mean death is the only option:

I wanted to write this book to encourage other men, the same way I was encouraged to get tested early, without it, my life might not have been saved. I believe that the thought of having Prostate Cancer and the overall stigma that comes along with it, including condemnation of sexual deficiencies, is enough to scare a lot of men out of even having the conversation about prostate health in general. Cancer is a life threatening disease, which means that death is a possibility, but that doesn't mean death is the only option.

You are bigger than Prostate Cancer, and even the idea that you might one day get it. Do not let it take you mentally. Life is still an option if you are willing to take the necessary steps to ensure yearly screenings and to get treatment if it becomes necessary. God too has healing power, and with his grace, I continue to go on with my life, reach my dreams, and enjoy my family. I have five grandchildren, and one God grandchild now. I enjoy watching them grow up. Love teaching them yoga, chess, tennis and golf is a joy that I won't ever take for granted. I am sixty-six still running behind my younger grandkids.

# Advice to you:

It's important to stay focused on your health of course, but also not letting your dreams go untended to as well. I had to continue with my dream as a real estate investor.

I renovated homes, and rented out clean affordable housing to people who needed them. Focused on my Spiritual growth, my family, hobbies and businesses allowed me to keep some sort of normalcy in my life during that devastating time, and I would suggest that you try to keep as much normalcy as you can as well.

African-American men are more prone to Prostate Cancer because of the pigmentation of their skin. We absorb Vitamin D from the sun better, having been brought to America where the sun is less intense causes a deficiency thus more likely producing Prostate Cancer. We know that the American high-fat diet feeds the mutated gene (abnormal gene) that begins to grow into a cancer tumor. Men who have high levels of testosterone (male hormone) that feeds this tumor also. If you are an African American male, you should talk to your doctor about getting tested at forty instead of the nationally recommended age of fifty. There is nothing taboo about wanting to live for you, and your loved ones. Again, awareness is our first line of defense against this disease.

We know that the American high-fat diet feeds the mutated gene (abnormal gene) that begins to grow into a cancer tumor. Men who have high levels of testosterone (male hormone) that feeds this tumor also. If you are an African American male, you should talk to your doctor about getting tested at forty instead of the nationally recommended age of fifty. There is nothing taboo about wanting to live for you, and your loved ones. Again, awareness is our first line of defense against this disease.

Whether you are a cancer survivor or someone who just wants to prevent any number of diseases, PCFs - The Science of Living Well, Beyond Cancer Foundation, is an invaluable resource. One in three people will be diagnosed with some form of cancer in their lifetime. Most of us know someone with cancer, but we all wish we didn't. An aging population combined with poor lifestyle choices has resulted in an overall rise in chronic disease, including cancer, diabetes, heart disease, autoimmune disease, and depression. The good news is that 42% of cancer is thought to be preventable. You can become a participant in your own health outcomes with a few simple lifestyle suggestions in this guide. You can inherit from either parent it is important to know the health history of your mother's father and brothers too because you can get this gene from your mother's side of the family or your father's side. You must know both family's health history and if someone in your family has or had Prostate Cancer. If it was detected in their fifties, there's a chance that you may have the gene that causes Prostate Cancer also. It's best to be screened as early as age forty. For Caucasian and Asian men should be screened for prostate cancer starting at age fifty.

If Prostate Cancer raises its ugly head in African- American men, it is more aggressive. We are not exactly sure why, but we know high levels of the male hormone testosterone are one of the reasons. We must find this cancer as soon as possible in its early stages. When it is found in its early stages. found it is not deadly and it is curable, I am a witness. We now know that certain chemicals, herbicide and insecticides can cause cancer, namely Agent Orange, this is why some of the veterans who were exposed to Agent Orange had a higher rate of prostate cancer.

When I had my biopsy at age fifty-two my PSA was 3.6, which was considered low risk for cancer. Every man should have his gene tested for Prostate Cancer; this will give you a heads-up to let you know that you have the gene. If you do, you must be very vigilant in getting a PSA screen for Prostate Cancer as early as possible and have it checked yearly. We now know

## CANCER WINNER

that the earlier we find this cancer, and treat it, it is curable. You do not have to die from Prostate Cancer if caught early. Early detection plays a huge role in getting started on treatments that could save your life.

# Following is information about available treatment for Prostate Cancer

# Final Thoughts

As I write the final chapter of my book we are now in the midst of a global pandemic, COVID-19. Many have died, as scientists and doctors around the globe search for a vaccine for this horrible virus. Scientists dealing with COVID-19 are talking about testing vaccines through clinical trials. This will require many volunteers. Prostate cancer researchers and doctors are also testing new drugs and procedures for the treatment of prostate cancer. In order to do this, they also need the participation of volunteers. Not only can testing and clinical research save the lives of those we love, but it can save many generations of men who would not be here without some type of treatment to prolong the lives of those diagnosed. Particularly, generations in the African-American community, because we die at an alarming rate compared to other races.

I am fortunate, my cancer was caught very early, and we were able to treat it in its early stages, thank God. I went in for screening every year starting at age thirty-five, now I am sixty-six years of age and cancer-free for fourteen years my PSA is non- detectable .01 Thank God for that. Had I not stayed on top of it, got screened every year, had a PSA, blood work, and a digital rectal exam who knows we may not have found the cancer until it was in its late stages. I would've been in "big trouble" according to my doctor. So, you see regular screening is a must.

# Acknowledgments

This book has taken me more than ten years to prepare and four years to write. There were many people in my life who encouraged me during this entire process. There were times where it didn't seem like I would ever get through it, but with persistence and a keen focus, I was finally able to complete my dream of writing this book for the many men who need this knowledge through hearing my story. I want to thank everyone who participated, helped, and supported me throughout this journey. Without this, this project would not be possible. Nothing in life is ever successful without the collaborative effort of many gifted people. Thank you to those who were a witness to the production of this project, and those who were willing to network and submit their talent, experience, and passion for a common goal of mine getting this information written. I am always reminded that we are the total of all the people we have known, met, and learned from. This book is the product of several individuals whose are thoughts, ideas perspectives, and work have given me the exposure and knowledge I have placed in this book. I wish to thank my wife Doris, our children Malcolm and Katrina, and our six grandchildren: Spell Adera, Joshua, Myles, Braxton and Noah; and Lil Katrina, for their patience and understanding during this process. Your support through what felt like endless days and nights trying to get this information will forever be appreciated. To all my friends, family and family in Christ, thank you for all your input, and never-ending support. My pastor,  , I want to thank him for praying with me, encouraging me and referring me Dr. Walsh. To Martha Dixon who encouraged and pushed me to get this book completed And all the guys who have experienced prostate cancer or who are going through Prostate Cancer, I have read some of your develop and define these ideas and concepts, sharing your experiences gave me an unforgettable force to write this book.

## Types of treatments

The treatments for prostate cancer depend on several factors, including the stage and aggressi-veness of the cancer, as well as the overall health and preferences of the patient. Here are some common treatments for prostate cancer: Active Surveillance: In some cases, especially for early-stage and slow-growing prostate cancer, active surveillance may be recommended. This approach involves closely monitoring the cancer through regular check-ups, prostate specific antigens (PSA) are signs of disease progression.

## Surgery

The most common surgical treatment for prostate cancer is a radical prostatectomy, which involves the removal of the entire prostate gland. This procedure can be done through open surgery or minimally invasive techniques, such as laparoscopic or roboticassisted surgery.

## Radiation Therapy

This treatment involves using high-energy X-rays or other forms of radiation to destroy cancer cells or inhibit their growth. External beam radiation therapy (EBRT) delivers radiation from outside the body, while brachytherapy involves placing radioactive implants directly into the prostate. Radiation therapy may be used as the primary treatment or in combination with surgery or other treatments.

# Hormone Therapy

Prostate cancer is often fueled by male hormones, particularly testosterone. Hormone therapy aims to suppress or block the production or action of these hormones, slowing down the growth of cancer cells. It can be done through medications (such as luteinizing hormone-releasing hormone agonists or anti-androgens) or through surgical removal of the testicles (orchiectomy).

# Chemotherapy

Chemotherapy drugs can be used to treat advanced prostate cancer that has spread to other parts of the body. Chemotherapy is typically given intravenously and works by targeting and killing rapidly dividing cancer cells throughout the body.

# Therapy

Targeted therapy drugs specifically target certain molecules or pathways involved in the growth and survival of cancer cells. They can be used to treat advanced prostate cancer that has become resistant to hormone therapy. Examples of targeted therapies for prostate cancer include abiraterone and enzalutamide.

# Immunotherapy

Immunotherapy helps to stimulate the body's immune system to recognize and attack cancer cells. Some immunotherapy drugs, such as sepulture-T, have been approved for the treatment of advanced prostate cancer. It's important to note that the choice of treatment depends on individual circumstances, and a comprehensive evaluation by a healthcare professional is necessary to determine the most appropriate treatment plan.

# Laser treatment

As an alternative to conventional treat- ments, laser treatment is an innovative strategy being investigated for prostate cancer. Prostate cancer is treated mostly with two types of laser-based therapies.

# Laser Ablation

This method, sometimes referred to as laser ablation therapy or laser interstitial thermal therapy (LITT), uses laser radiationto heat and eliminate prostate malignant tissue. The rectum or perineum—the space between the scrotum and anus—is utilized to introduce a thin laser fiber into the prostate. The laser is then used to precisely and carefully burn the tumor. The heat kills the cancer cells while causing the least amount of harm to the surrounding healthy tissue.

# Photodynamic Therapy (PDT)

PDT is a medical procedure that combines the use of a laser light source and a photosensitizing medication. After being injected into the circulation, laser light is focused on the prostate, the photosensitizing medication builds up in malignant cells. After that, a certain wavelength of laser light is focused on the prostate, activating the photosensitizing medication and producing reactive oxygen species that kill the cancer cells.

Compared to surgery or radiation therapy, laser therapies provide several potential benefits, such as minimum invasiveness, accurate targeting, quicker recovery periods, and a lower risk of problems. It is noteworthy, although, that laser treatments for prostate cancer are still regarded as investigational or experimental, and clinical trials are still being conducted to assess their long-term safety and efficacy.

Usually, these treatments are provided as part of clinical research studies and in specialist facilities. It's important to speak with a medical expert who specializes in this field if you or someone you know is thinking about laser treatment for prostate cancer. They can go over the possible advantages, risks, and best available treatments.

# Rates of anxiety

For a variety of reasons, men who receive a prostate cancer diagnosis may see a considerable increase in anxiety. When receiving a diagnosis, patients may feel anxious as they await test results and consider the likelihood of developing cancer. Worries over the possible adverse effects and extended consequences of treatments such as radiation therapy or surgery can also induce anxiety during the decision making phase. Handling sexual function changes brought on by therapy can make anxiety worse, which can be detrimental to relationships and one's sense of value. People may feel alone even after a successful course of treatment because of the stigma associated with being diagnosed with cancer. Anxiety significantly lowers one's overall quality of life by lowering social and physical interactions, producing despair, and interfering with sleep. Anxiety significantly lowers a person's overall quality of life by affecting treatment decisions, decreasing social and physical activities, lowering sleep quality, and producing sadness. Psychological therapy like counseling, in addition to support from family, friends, and medical professionals, is very helpful in managing anxiety. More and more preventive actions are being taken, such as giving patients tools to help them cope with their anxiety and offering guidance and instruction through the diagnosis process. Recognizing and treating anxiety is essential because, with the right support and treatments, it may be managed, substan-tially improving a patient's mental well-being during the prostate cancer treatment process.

# Disease Stage

Depending on the stage of the disease at that point, men with prostate cancer frequently experience varied degrees of worry following their diagnosis. People who have localized or early-stage prostate cancer may experience anxiety related to the uncertainty around the illness's progress and the potential outcomes of different treatment options. Fear of the unknown, which includes concerns about possible adverse effects and the long-term repercussions of particular treatments, can frequently be the root cause of anxiety. However, anxiety levels may rise in those who have been told they have advanced or metastatic prostate cancer. Patients may experience more stress and worry when they have to deal with a more complex treatment plan and more challenges in managing their condition. They may also perceive the disease as being more severe and conscious of potential impacts on their general health. To tailor interventions and support to the specific needs of individuals at different phases of their prostate cancer journey, it is imperative to recognize the changes in anxiety levels according to the disease's stage.

## Treatment Options

When men are diagnosed with prostate cancer, their anxiety levels are significantly impacted by the variety of treatment options available. When it comes to choosing a course of therapy, people often experience anxiety while carefully weighing the pros and cons of each option. The specifics of treatment regimens, such as hormone therapy, radiation therapy, and surgery, add a complex web of factors. Anxiety can arise from worries about the short and long term negative consequences, functional changes, and quality-of-life implications of these treatments. When presented with these alternatives, patients frequently experience anxiety, so healthcare providers must provide comprehensive information and support to help people make decisions that are in keeping with their preferences and medical needs.

## Individual Characteristics

Depending greatly on their unique characteristics, men who receive a prostate cancer diagnosis face varying degrees of anxiety. Because older patients may have Ars worries and coping techniques than younger patients, age can have a significant effect on treatment outcomes. Previous experiences with cancer or chronic illness might either improve or worsen a person's capacity to deal with a new diagnosis. Individual coping methods and psychological resilience are also critical because those with effective support networks and stress management skills can also experience reduced anxiety. However, pre- existing mental health issues like depression or generalized anxiety disorder might exacerbate anxiety symptoms that follow a prostate cancer diagnosis. Targeted mental health therapies and support are required to guarantee comprehensive care and emotional well- being during the cancer experience. Understanding these distinctive characteristics is essential to adjusting medical care and other support to meet each person's specific needs.

# Fear of recurrence and progression

Anxiety among men with prostate cancer is primarily brought on by dread of the disease's advancement and recurrence. An individual's overall health may be significantly impacted by persistent concern and anxiety brought on by the uncertainty surrounding the likelihood of the disease spreading or returning. This dread often affects many aspects of day-to-day living, including decisions about medical care and follow-up as well as mental and psychological health. Patients may feel more stressed out managing the ongoing surveillance and monitoring that accompany a prostate cancer diagnosis. This highlights the need to receive comprehensive emotional and psychological care during the cancer journey to reduce worry and provide a sense of stability and control.

# Psychological Distress

Psychological distress is a prevalent and complex side effect of prostate cancer that plays a significant role in the anxiety experienced by persons with the disease. A sense of self-identity that is broken by the diagnosis, worry about changes in one's physical and sexual functioning and existential concerns about death and the purpose of life are just a few of the many causes that can trigger the distress. The financial strain of medical and treatment expenses, along with concerns about the illness's impact on social roles and interpersonal connections, exacerbates complex psychological discomfort. To help people overcome these challenges and improve their emotional health both during and after their journey with prostate cancer, a comprehensive psychosocial support and counseling program is essential. The combination of these upsetting elements can have a debilitating effect, increasing anxiety.

# Impact on Quality of Life

In actuality, a man's general quality of life may be significantly and permanently impacted by the In actuality, a man's general quality of life may be significantly and permanently impacted by the worry that follows a prostate cancer diagnosis. An individual's mental health is negatively impacted by persistent anxiety, which can lead to depressive symptoms and a decrease in general life satisfaction. Consequently, emotional health is often adversely affected. Relationship tension can result from anxiety's ability to obstruct communication and emotional connection with partners and loved ones. In addition to impairing sexual performance, the negative effects may result in low selfesteem and damaged relationships. Anxiety can also make it difficult for a person to psychologically adjust to their diagnosis and treatment plan, which can lead to feelings of helplessness and a loss of selfcontrol. Severe anxiety can hinder a person's ability to manage life's obstacles, reduce treatment adherence, and keep them from engaging in vital self-care activities. This highlights the significance of treating and managing anxiety for individuals with prostate cancer to preserve their overall quality of life.

## Addressing Anxiety

It is critical to recognize the incidence and impact of anxiety in men with prostate cancer to offer them the care and therapies they require. In addition to providing medical care, healthcare practitioners should adopt a multidisciplinary strategy that includes psychological and emotional assistance. This approach comprises early anxiety assessment, compassionate and clear communication of the diagnosis and possible treatments, and access to mental health professionals, such as psychologists or social workers, who specialize in cancer related anxiety. Support groups can provide a beneficial environment where individuals can share their stories and learn coping skills from others who have had similar challenges. Education and resources on stress reduction, relaxation methods, and anxiety management may also be helpful to patients and their families. By treating anxiety holistically, medical providers can enhance the overall health and quality of life of men who have been diagnosed with prostate cancer.

## Routine screening

Part of the follow-up therapy for patients with prostate cancer should indeed include routine screening for anxiety symptoms. Validated assessment tools like the Hospital Anxiety and Depression Scale (HADS) can offer systematic and standardized approaches to measuring anxiety levels. Through these assessments at key points throughout treatment and follow-up, clinicians can identify patients who may be severely anxious before symptoms spiral out of control. Early intervention and the beginning of tailored support are made possible by this proactive approach, which can greatly enhance patients' emotional health and anxiety management throughout their prostate cancer journey. It also makes it easier to track how anxiety evolves and adjust interventions as needed.

# Psychoeducation

Psychoeducation is a crucial component of anxiety management for men with prostate cancer. It comprises providing detailed and accurate information about the disease, available treatments, and potential side effects. By being informed about all the components of their diagnosis and the therapies that they might choose from, patients can make decisions that are consistent with their values and preferences. This knowledge helps reduce the uncertainty and dread that are often associated with prostate cancer by giving patients a sense of empowerment and control over their healthcare journey. It also establishes a collaborative relationship between patients and healthcare providers, facilitating open and effective communication that can further alleviate anxiety and promote a more collaborative and patient-focused treatment strategy. Ultimately, psychoeducation raises patients' psychological toughness and gives them information, which helps them feel better emotionally and live a better life during their prostate cancer journey.

# Psychosocial Support

Psychosocial support services are a crucial component of overall care for men with prostate cancer. Individual therapy, support groups, and online communities offer safe and caring environments where people can freely communicate their fears, share their stories, and get emotional support from others who understand their path. In addition to treating the physical elements of prostate cancer, these treatments also address the psychological and emotional fallout from the diagnosis. They provide helpful coping strategies for managing the psychological challenges associated with prostate cancer and help normalize anxiety, which reduces the sense of isolation that usually accompanies the disease. The feeling of community and shared experiences that these support groups promote may be a wonderful source of comfort and empowerment for people, and it can have a positive impact on their overall quality of life and mental well-being throughout and after their prostate cancer treatment journey.

# Cognitive-behavioral Therapy (CBT)

Cognitive-behavioral therapy (CBT) is a wellknown and scientifically validated therapeutic approach that is effective in treating anxiety and other emotional issues. When dealing with anxiety symptoms related to prostate cancer, cognitive behavioral therapy (CBT) therapies may be quite helpful. Cognitive behavioral therapy (CBT) focuses on identifying and challenging negative beliefs and behaviors to swap them out with more adaptable and useful mental processes. It also emphasizes the need to develop coping mechanisms, which enable people to handle anxiety-provoking situations more adeptly. Cognitive behavioral therapy (CBT) has been shown to significantly reduce anxiety and enhance overall well- being in men going through this challenging time by promoting emotional regulation and providing tailored tools to handle the specific stresses that come with a prostate cancer diagnosis. Its versatility and evidence- based approach make it a valuable tool for the psychological support and care of patients with prostate cancer.

# Mindfulness-based interventions

More people are realizing the advantages of mindfulness- based therapy for improving overall well-being and lowering anxiety in prostate cancer patients. These therapies, such as mindfulness-based stress reduction (MBSR) and mindfulness meditation, emphasize accepting oneself without criticizing one's thoughts and feelings and cultivating present-moment awareness.

By practicing mindfulness, patients might learn to notice their worry without passing judgment on it and build emotional resilience. People may thus feel less anxious and find it simpler to cope with the psychological repercussions of prostate cancer. Mindfulness-based interventions offer helpful strategies for lowering stress, enhancing emotional regulation, and cultivating a sense of control in a situation that often feels overwhelming. These techniques help people deal with prostate cancer in a more calm and emotionally balanced way.

# Genetic Susceptibility

Research has indicated that African American men are more genetically predisposed to prostate cancer than males of Caucasian descent. The genetic markers linked to elevated risk, such as BRCA gene variations, will be covered in detail in this section along with how they may affect specific preventive and screening approaches.

## Variants in the BRCA Gene

The well-known genes BRCA1 and BRCA2 are linked to ovarian and breast cancer syndromes that run in families. Recent studies have revealed that some variations of these genes are also associated with a higher risk of prostate cancer, especially in men who identify as African-American. According to studies, African American men who carry these mutations in the BRCA gene are two to three times more likely than those who do not to develop prostate cancer.

## Implications for Targeted Prevention

Strategies for targeted prevention could benefit from the discovery of BRCA gene variations in African-American men. Screening for prostate cancer earlier and more frequently may be beneficial for those who have these variations. According to National Comprehensive Cancer Network (NCCN) guidelines, African American men with BRCA gene variations or a family history of prostate cancer should think about prostate cancer screening at a younger age (e.g., 40–45 years). Better treatment outcomes may result from early detection.

## Implications of Targeted Screening

Digital rectal examination (DRE) and prostate specific antigen (PSA) testing are commonly used in the screening process for prostate cancer. Nonetheless, more screening methods could be required given that African-American men have BRCA gene variations. For example, in men with

BRCA2 mutations, multiparametric magnetic resonance imaging (MRI) of the prostate has demonstrated potential in identifying aggressive prostate cancer. In this high risk group, combining MRI with conventional screening techniques may increase the precision of prostate cancer detection.

## Prospects for Precision Medicine

The discovery that African American men with prostate cancer had BRCA gene mutations provides opportunities for precision medicine techniques. In patients with BRCA gene mutations, targeted treatments such as poly (ADP-ribose) polymerase (PARP) inhibitors have been approved for the treatment of advanced prostate cancer. Therefore, discovering these mutations can aid in directing therapy choices and enhancing prognoses for African-American males suffering from prostate cancer.

## Genetic Counseling and Testing

These are essential given the effects of BRCA gene variations on prostate cancer risk and treatment. Individuals and families can learn about the genetic foundation of prostate cancer, the possible dangers linked to particular gene variants, and the available alternatives for treatment and prevention through genetic counseling. The identification of those who might profit from focused screening and therapies can be aided by genetic testing.

## Research and Future Directions

To fully comprehend the range of genetic factors influencing the differences in prostate cancer incidence between African-American and Caucasian males, more research is required. Finding more genetic markers linked to higher risk can improve models used to assess risk and provide guidance for targeted screening and preventive measures. Research in this area must be advanced by collaboration between academics, medical professionals, and the African-American community to translate results into clinical practice.

Overall, African-American males are more likely to develop prostate cancer due to genetic factors, such as the existence of specific BRCA gene mutations. Precision medicine, early screening, and targeted prevention are made possible by our growing understanding of these genetic variables. Identifying high risk people and directing appropriate interventions can be facilitated by integrating genetic counseling and testing into clinical practice. To decrease prostate cancer disparities among varied populations and enhance our understanding of genetic vulnerability, more research in this area is required.

Prostate cancer is a significant health concern, and there are observed differences in its prevalence, incidence, and outcomes among various racial and ethnic groups, including African American men.

# Learning from my experience

## Higher Incidence and Mortality Rates:

African American men have the highest incidence rate of prostate cancer among all racial and ethnic groups in the United States. They also experience a higher mortality rate compared to other groups.

## Younger Age of Onset:

Prostate cancer tends to occur at a younger age in African American men compared to other ethnic groups. This means that they are often diagnosed at more advanced stages of the disease.

## Aggressive Tumor Types:

African American men are more likely to develop aggressive types of prostate cancer, which may contribute to the higher mortality rates. Studies have shown that they have a higher prevalence of Gleason score 8-10 tumors, which are associated with a poorer prognosis.

## Access to Healthcare:

Disparities in healthcare access and utilization may contribute to differences in prostate cancer outcomes. African American men may face barriers such as lower rates of health insurance coverage, less frequent prostate cancer screening, and delayed access to medical care.

## Genetic Factors:

Genetic factors may play a role in the disparities observed in prostate cancer. Some studies suggest a genetic predis- position among African American men that may contribute to the develoment of more aggressive forms of the disease.

## Socioeconomic Factors:

Socioeconomic factors, including income and education levels, can influence health outcomes. African American men may be disproportionately affected by socioeconomic disparities, impacting their ability to access quality healthcare.

## Biological Factors:

There is ongoing research to understand whether there are biological factors that contribute to the higher prevalence and aggressiveness of prostate cancer in African American men. Some studies suggest that there may be genetic or hormonal factors involved.

## Awareness and Screening Practices:

Differences in awareness and adherence to prostate cancer screening guidelines may contribute to the observed disparities. African American men may be less likely to undergo regular screening, leading to later-stage diagnoses. One of the most common cancers impacting men globally is prostate cancer. Surgery, radiation therapy, chemotherapy, and hormone therapy are common treatments for prostate cancer. Among the many adverse effects of these medicines are erectile and sexual dysfunction. To address these adverse effects and enhance general wellbeing, many patients and healthcare professionals investigate complementary approaches. Prostate massage is among these methods. This essay will examine the potential advantages and drawbacks of prostate massage as a supplemental treatment for people with prostate cancer.

# Prostate cancer and massage therapy:

The manual stimulation of the prostate gland, which is situated directly beneath the bladder, is the purpose of prostate massage. Prostate massage should only be taken into consideration after speaking with a healthcare provider, especially in the case of prostate cancer. Prostate massage, which is usually administered by a licensed healthcare professional, may benefit people with prostate cancer in a number of ways.

## Relieving Urinary Symptoms:

Urinary problems including incontinence and retention can be brought on by prostate cancer and its therapies. Prostate massage has the potential to mitigate these symptoms by improving urine flow and easing associated discomfort.

## Enhanced Sexual Function:

After receiving treatment, many men with prostate cancer still struggle with infidelity. Enhancing sexual satisfaction and maybe contributing to and maybe contributing to the restorati on of sexual function is the use of prostate massage to increase blood flow to the area.

## Prostate Health:

By assisting in the clearance of prostatic ducts and so lowering the risk of infection and inflammation, regular prostate massage may benefit prostate health.

## Stress Reduction:

Patients with prostate cancer may experience emotional and psychological difficulties. When done in a secure and encouraging setting, prostate massage may help lower tension and anxiety levels.

## Safety and Requirements:

It is imperative to stress that prostate massage ought to be contemplated only following a comprehensive consultation with a medical professional, ideally one with expertise in prostate health. There are a few crucial factors and safety measures to remember:

## Professional Advice

A licensed healthcare practitioner with experience performing prostate massages should be the ones administering the treatment. It is never appropriate for patients to try to massage their prostates on their own.

## Medical History:

To guarantee the safety and suitability of the procedure, healthcare professionals should be aware of the patient's medical history, including any prior prostate disorders or treatments.

## Informed Consent:

Before giving their permission for a prostate massage, patients should be fully informed about the technique, its possible advantages, and any hazards involved.

## Comfort and Privacy:

To guarantee the patient's calmness during the process, a nurturing and comfortable setting should be offered. During the procedure, communication and privacy are crucial.

# Frequent Monitoring:

If prostate massage is advised, it should be performed as part of a thorough treatment plan and under regular observation by a medical professional. Patients with prostate cancer who are experiencing problems with their urine and erection may find some relief and potential advantages from prostate massage, which is a complimentary method. But it's important to proceed cautiously with this treatment, consulting with skilled medical professionals who focus on prostate health for advice. Traditional medical therapies for prostate cancer should not be replaced by prostate massage; rather, it should be viewed as one component of an all- encompassing therapy approach. Prostate massage may improve the quality of life for patients with prostate cancer, but its application will be guided by a deeper comprehension of its possible advantages and disadvantages as this field of study develops.

# 20 of The Most Common Questions and Answer About Prostate Cancer

# 1. Question:

What's driving the racial disparities surrounding prostate cancer diagnoses and survival rates?

# Answer:

Studies suggest there's probably a genetic factor that results in Black men having higher diagnosis rates than men of other backgrounds. We are still attempting to understand this.

# 2. Question:

Do you believe prostate cancer is a taboo preventing people from discussing it?

# Answer:

Absolutely. As Black men, we keep things close to the hip. In addition, the history of mistreatment of African Americans in general and within the medical field, such as the Tuskegee experiment, there is a lack of trust in the healthcare system. Some men don't want to receive a PSA because they may be diagnosed with cancer and they think back to the experiences of their fathers or uncles with prostate cancer when treatment was more likely to cause complications such as incontinence and impotence. It became the brand, even though the technology has greatly improved, and complications are not as bad as 30 years ago. As we educate men, we demonstrate that technology has improved and treatment options have fewer risks, while highlighting that men diagnosed with prostate cancer are living a normal lifestyle. This information will change the conversation.

# 3. Question:

At what age should African American men get screened?

# Answer:

Men at the age of 40 should discuss the advantages and limitations of screening with their healthcare provider.

## 4. Question:

How can I reduce my risk?

## Answer:

While there are some risks you can't take, like your age, there are some strategies you can take to reduce your risk of prostate cancer or catch it early to achieve better outcomes for your health.

•    Change your lifestyle: Avoid smoking if you are a smoker. Quitting smoking may reduce the severity of prostate cancer or reduce its severity. Furthermore, maintain a healthy weight.

•    Consider screening: Talk to your healthcare provider about the advantages and disadvantages of prostate cancer screening.

•    If you are Black, or if you have a close relative (father, son, or brother) who had prostate cancer before age 65, start talking to your healthcare provider about prostate cancer when you are 45. If more than one close relative had prostate cancer before 65 years old, have that conversation at age 40.

## 5. Question:

What is the most common cause of prostate cancer?

## Answer:

The American Cancer Society's estimates for prostate cancer in the United States for 2024 are:

•    About 299,010 new cases of prostate cancer.

•    About 35,250 deaths from prostate cancer.

The number of prostate cancers diagnosed each year decreased significantly from 2007 to 2014, resulting in fewer men being screened due to changes in screening recommendations. Since 2014, the incidence rate has increased by 3% per year and by around 5% per year for advanced-stage prostate cancer.

# 6. Question:

How difficult is being diagnosed with Prostate Cancer?

# Answer:

The second-leading cause of cancer death in American men have prostate cancer, with only lung cancer is the primary cause. About 1 in 44 men will die of prostate cancer.

Prostate cancer can be a serious disease, but most men who are diagnosed with prostate cancer do not die from it. More than 3.3 million men in the United States who have been diagnosed with prostate cancer at some point are still alive today.

The prostate cancer death rate declined by about half from 1993 to 2013, most likely due to earlier detection and advances in treatment. In recent years, the death rate has stabilized, likely reflecting the rise in cancers being found at an advanced stage.

# 7. Question:

Is genetics a factor in prostate cancer?

# Answer:

In addition, new research on gene changes in prostate cancer cells enables scientists to better understand how prostate cancer develops. This could also assist in designing medicines to target these changes. Learning more about these gene changes might be helpful in other ways as well, such as:

• Identifying which men are most likely to develop (or already have) prostate cancer.

• Determining which men might need a second prostate biopsy, even if an initial biopsy doesn't find cancer.

• Determining which prostate cancers are Screening for prostate cancer is as simple as contacting your primary care physician, discussing your family history with him or her, and having a PSA blood test. This test may be conducted during a regular physical or wellness visit. Shared decision making between physician and patient is crucial to discuss your risk, your need for testing, and the next steps to take if your PSA level is elevated and concerning. Knowing your risk can save your life (and therefore should be treated)

• Determining if specific treatments such as newer targeted therapy drugs might be helpful.

• Identifying which men might benefit from genetic testing to see if they inherited a gene change (and therefore might have a higher risk for other cancers as well)

# 8. Question:

What are some ways I can prevent prostate cancer?

# Answer:

The effects of body weight, physical activity, and diet for prostate cancer are not completely clear, but there are ways you can reduce your risk.

Some studies have suggested that men with excessive body weight have a greater risk of developing advanced prostate cancer or prostate cancer that is more likely to be fatal.

Although not all studies agree, some have found a higher risk of prostate cancer in men who consume dairy products and calcium.

For now, the best advice about diet and activity to possibly reduce the risk of prostate cancer is to:

• Get to and stay at a healthy weight.

- Be physically active.

- Follow a healthy eating pattern, which includes a variety of colorful fruits and vegetables and whole grains, and avoid or limit red and processed meats, sugar sweetened beverages, and highly processed foods.

It may be beneficial to limit calcium supplements and not consume too much calcium in the diet. This does not indicate that men who are being treated for prostate cancer should not take calcium supplements if their doctor recommends them.

# 9. Question:

What should my PSA level be?

# Answer:

According to pubmed.ncbi.nlm.nih.gov, the following are the normal reference ranges for serum prostate-specific antigen (PSA) in black men based on their sample 95th percentiles:

- 40–49 years old: 0–1.9 ng/mL
- 50–59 years old: 3.8 ng/mL
- 60–69 years old: 5.7 ng/mL

According to pubmed.ncbi.nlm.nih.gov, the following are normal reference ranges for PSA in black men:

- 40s: 0–2.0 ng/mL
- 50s: 0–4.0 ng/mL
- 60s: 0–4.5 ng/mL

According to the American Cancer Society, normal PSA levels range from 0 to 4 ng/mL. Levels below 2.5 ng/mL are considered safe and those PSA levels over 4.0 ng/mL require further testing or monitoring.

## 10. Question:

Is it difficult to get screened for Prostate Cancer?

## Answer:

Screening for prostate cancer is as simple as contacting your primary care physician, discussing your family history with him or her, and having a PSA blood test. This test may be conducted during an annual physical or wellness visit. Shared decision making between physician and patient is crucial to discuss your risk, your need for testing, and the next steps to take if your PSA level is elevated and concerning. Knowing your risk can save your life.

## 11. Question:

What is the cause of Prostate Cancer?

## Answer:

It's unclear what causes prostate cancer. Doctors are aware that prostate cancer begins when cells in the prostate develop changes in their DNA. A cell's DNA contains instructions that tell a cell what to do. The changes indicate that the cells will grow and divide more rapidly than normal cells do. The abnormal cells continue living when other cells die.

The accumulating abnormal cells create a tumor that can spread to nearby tissue. Over time, some abnormal cells can break apart and spread (metastasize) to other parts of the body.

## 12. Question:

What are some complications associated with Prostate Cancer?

## Answer:

Complications of prostate cancer and its treatments include:

- Cancer that spreads (metastasizes). Prostate cancer can spread to nearby organs, such as your bladder, or travel through your bloodstream or lymphatic system to your bones or other organs. Prostate cancer that is spread to the bones can cause pain and broken bones. Once prostate cancer has spread to other areas of the body, it may still respond to treatment and may be controlled, but it's unlikely to be cured.

- Incontinence. Both prostate cancer and its treatment can result in urinary incontinence. Treatment for incontinence depends on the type you have; how severe it is and the likelihood it will improve over time. Treatment options may include medications, catheters, and surgery.

- Erectile dysfunction. Erectile dysfunction can result from prostate cancer or its treatment, including surgery, radiation, or hormone treatments. Medications, vacuum devices that assist in achieving erection, and surgery are available to treat erectile dysfunction.

## 13. Question:

Where does prostate cancer spread?

## Answer:

Prostate cancer can be spread to the lymph nodes and bones most often. It can also be transmitted to other organs such as the liver or lungs. Cancer cells disintegrate from the tumor in the prostate and travel through the lymphatic system or bloodstream to other areas. When prostate cancer is spread to other parts of the body, it usually occurs in the bones first. These areas may cause pain and weak bones that may break. The most prevalent symptoms of metastatic prostate cancer are swelling and pain around the area where the cancer has spread. Cancer cells can prevent lymph fluid from draining away, which may cause swelling in the legs due to fluid buildup in that area. In many cases, prostate cancer is relatively slow to develop, which means that it can take years to become large enough to be detected, and even longer to be metastasized outside the prostate.

## 14. Question:

How quickly does prostate cancer usually spread?

## Answer:

In many cases, prostate cancer is relatively slow-growing, which means that it can take years to become large enough to be detected, and even longer to be metastasized outside of the prostate. However, some cases are more aggressive and require more urgent intervention.

When a man is diagnosed with prostate cancer, his treatment team will evaluate his cancer and his overall health to create a treatment plan that will give him the greatest chance of defeating the cancer. Treatment can range from a wait and watch approach to a very aggressive medical and surgical plan.

## 15. Question:

Is it possible to have a high PSA and not have prostate cancer?

## Answer:

Besides cancer, other conditions that can raise PSA levels include an enlarged prostate prostate (also known as benign prostatic hyperplasia or BPH) and an inamed or infected prostate (prostatitis).

## 16. Question:

Are PSA results ever incorrect?

## Answer:

According to previous studies conducted in clinical trials, 10–12% of men who undergo regular PSA testing will experience a false positive outcome. False positive results can have a significant impact on the clinical management and outcome of the patient, particularly due to potential adverse effects related to the diagnostic process (biopsy, surgery, and treatment). Biopsies, for instance, can cause infections as well as serious complications such as urinary incontinence and sexual intercourse.

# 17. Question:

What are some symptoms of Prostate Cancer?

# Answer:

- Difficulty starting urination.
- Weak or interrupted urine flow.
- Urinating often, especially at night.

- Trouble emptying the bladder completely.
- Pain or burning during urination.
- Blood in the urine or semen.
- Painful ejaculation.
- Dribbling of urine.
- Frequent pain or stiffness in the lower back, hips, pelvic or rectal area, or upper thighs.

# 18. Question:

Does stress increase the risk of Prostate Cancer?

# Answer:

While stress may not directly cause prostate issues, long term stress can weaken the immune system, alter your hormonal balance, and make you more susceptible to disease. Meditation is a great way to ease daily stress and can also help you improve your mental health.

## 19. Question:

What happens during screening?

## Answer:

A PSA test involves having your blood drawn and sent to a laboratory for testing. Your doctor may also manually examine your prostate. He or she will keep you informed about the results and any next steps needed. If your doctor is concerned that you might have prostate cancer based on your PSA level or a manual exam, a biopsy to remove a small amount of tissue from the prostate will be the next step. This is the only way to test for the presence of cancer.

Although a PSA test is used mainly to evaluate prostate cancer, the results may be used to guide treatment recommendations if cancer is detected. Your PSA test may help determine how advanced a cancer is and after treatment, PSA levels can help determine if treatment was successful.

## 20. Question:

Is there a way to determine if my prostate cancer is aggressive?

## Answer:

The next step is to determine the level of aggressiveness (grade) of the cancer cells. A physician in a laboratory examines a sample of your cancer cells to determine how much cancer cells differ from the healthy cells. A higher grade indicates a more aggressive cancer that is more likely to spread quickly. Techniques used to determine aggressiveness of cancer include:

- Gleason score - The most common scale used to determine the grade of prostate cancer cells is called a Gleason score. Gleason scoring is a combination of two numbers and can range from 2 (nonaggressive cancer) to 10 (very aggressive cancer), though the lower portion of the range is not used as often. Most Gleason scores used to evaluate prostate biopsy samples range from 6 to 10. A score of 6 indicates that a low-grade prostate cancer is present. A score of 7 indicates a medium-grade prostate cancer. Scores from 8 to 10 indicate high-grade cancers.

## CANCER WINNER

- Genomic testing - Genomic testing analyzes your prostate cancer cells to determine which genes are present. This type of test can provide you with more information about your diagnosis. But it's not clear who might benefit most from this information, so the tests aren't widely used. Genomic tests are not necessary for every individual with prostate cancer, but they may provide more information for making treatment decisions in certain circumstances.

# CANCER WINNER